CW00517192

How to Analyze People

The guide to analyzing and influencing anyone by reading body language and reading people fast. How to connect with anyone, communicate effectively, develop deep relationships.

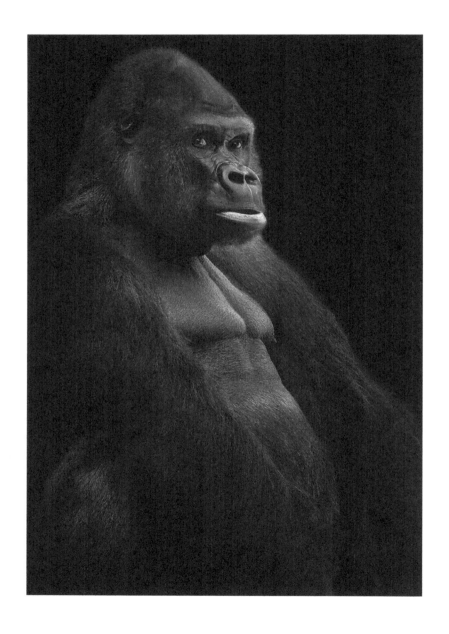

Table of Contents

The information in the following pages is broadly considered a truthful and accurate account of facts and as such, any inattention, use, or misuse of the information in question by the reader will render any resulting actions solely under their purview. There are no scenarios in which the publisher or the original author of this work can be in any fashion deemed liable for any hardship or damages that may befall them after undertaking information described herein.

Additionally, the information in the following pages is intended only for informational purposes and should thus be thought of as universal. As befitting its nature, it is presented without assurance regarding its prolonged validity or interim quality. Trademarks that are mentioned are done without written consent and can in no way be considered an endorsement from the trademark holder.

Introduction

Congratulations on purchasing this book and thank you for doing so.

The human body language is a remarkable thing. It can speak louder than words ever could and deliver messages so impactful when we are at a loss for words. Our bodies give out cues when we love someone, when we hate them, feel angry, when we are sad, happy, and more. It reveals all our innermost thoughts, feelings, desires, moods, and personalities. Whether we realize it or not, our bodies are constantly giving the people around us a glimpse of what may be happening on the inside.

Each day, our body gives out signals throughout the day which reflect the moods we're currently experiencing. It also reflects the situation that we find ourselves in. Without saying a word, our bodies allow others to read and - for the perceptive ones - form a hypothesis about what we may be experiencing or feeling right at that moment. This is called analyzing others, and this is why you've found yourself picking up this book. Because you *want* to better understand the people around you, to get a deeper glimpse into what might be going on.

Over the years, there has been a growing appreciation for the importance of learning how to analyze others. Each chapter of this book is going to address the eight key elements that you must understand in order to *better your understanding* of others. One gesture doesn't just reveal one type of message. Given the context and circumstance, that same gesture could hold several other meanings, and that is what makes body language and learning how to analyze others such an intriguing subject.

There are plenty of books on this subject on the market. Thanks again for choosing this one! Every effort was made to ensure it is full of as much useful information as possible. Please enjoy!

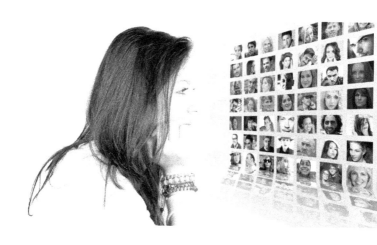

Chapter 1: Knowing Me, Knowing You

It is an intriguing prospect, isn't it? The idea that you could precisely decipher how and what someone is saying without them having to utter a word? The second body language that they are giving off which others might miss. But not you. Because you're perceptive, and you know exactly what to look for when you begin analyzing someone.

When was the last time you stopped to analyze yourself, though?

Before you can begin analyzing someone else, you need to learn how to analyze yourself first. Self-awareness is one of the core principles and a sign that someone possesses emotional intelligence. This key trait is what helps you understand who you are as a person. What your beliefs and your values are as well as the way that you react and respond to others.

When you look at yourself in the mirror, how well do you know the person who is looking back at you? Learning to analyze people is an important skill to have because it can help you strengthen the relationships that you have with them. But there is one relationship you need to work on strengthening first - *the relationship with yourself.*

Why It Is Important to Understand Yourself Before You Can Analyze Others

If you don't learn how to recognize and identify with yourself, you'll never be able to do that with others, too. At least, not entirely. When you're attempting to learn how to analyze someone else, you're attempting to look for clues which will be indicators about who they are and what they're feeling. However, it is equally important to do the same thing with yourself. When you're looking for clues as to why people react the way that they do, you also need to look for clues about why *you* react the way that you do. Only when you understand yourself entirely, can you then begin to understand others.

To understand and build better connections with the people around you, you need to first understand yourself. If you don't have the necessary self-awareness to begin understanding why you do or say the things that you do, how can you begin to understand someone else's intentions and where they're coming from? Remember, someone else could be reading and assessing your body language, too. Analyzing you the way you may be doing to them. What message do you want them to read?

So, if self-reflection is so important, why don't more people do it? There could be several reasons for that, including:

- **They're Unsure about What Needs to Be Done.** Many people don't necessarily spend enough time in self-reflection because they're simply unsure about what needs to be done. We are quick to analyze others, but when it comes to ourselves, that's where many fall short.

- **They Don't Particularly Enjoy It.** Self-reflection is not always the easiest process, especially because it forces people to confront all the emotions and thoughts that they would prefer to ignore. In fact, it is one of the most difficult skills to master personally. Weaknesses, vulnerability, fears, and more are all the emotions that many people prefer to keep buried or hidden, and self-reflection is a process that is going to force all these unpleasant qualities to the surface, which is why many people don't enjoy this process. For many people, acknowledging the flaws is the most difficult part of the process. Nobody likes to admit they've got faults which they need to work on. Pride and ego get in the way. This is largely responsible for why many people suffer from denial, completely blind to their own faults.

- **They Don't Understand How It Can Help.** As people, we tend to be motivated to do something only if we can see what is in it for us. We need the motivation to get us to do something we may not necessarily like or enjoy. Only if we can clearly see the benefits do we then take action. This is why many people don't spend enough time self-reflecting, because they don't see how this process is going to help them. They don't view it as a good use of their time, especially when they have a busy schedule.

- **They Don't Have Time.** It's a common phrase that is uttered these days. *I don't have time.* There never seems to be enough time to get things done. To those who feel like they are constantly on the move from one task to the next, asking them to spend several minutes in quiet self-reflection doesn't make any sense because they don't see it as a good use of their time.

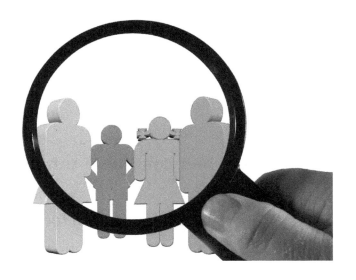

When you understand yourself and your personality a little better, you'll naturally become more understanding of others, too. If you notice the way that you behave and the body language signals that you emit, you'll be able to understand why someone else might be doing the same thing. If you're an introvert, for instance, you'll be able to acknowledge why other introverts may be displaying certain signals, because you will recognize them in yourself. It works the same way for extroverts, too. Understanding others begins, very simply, with understanding yourself first.

Self-Awareness and Emotional Intelligence

Human emotions remain the driving force of a lot of the things we say, think, and do. Emotions can be a very powerful, volatile force within us that may sometimes have difficulty trying to control. This is why emotional intelligence is linked to self-awareness. A clear sign that someone possesses a high level of emotional intelligence is when they can master and control not just their own emotions, but they can also exercise influence over the emotions of others, too.

Yes, emotional intelligence allows you to influence the way other people are feeling. In fact, you'll be able to understand the people around you even better when you've got emotional intelligence on your side. Made of five core principles, emotional intelligence involves self-awareness, self-reflection, motivation, social skills, and empathy. These five traits are the tools which are going to help you analyze others even better than ever because each of these qualities is working in a way that encourages you to be more observant about a person's body language.

Self-reflection, which is what this chapter has largely been focusing on, is first understanding your own emotions so you can then regulate your responses and reactions (self-regulation). To begin developing a deeper understanding of the people around you is where social skills and empathy come into play. Empathy is the ability to put yourself in someone else's shoes, to see things from their perspective, and to understand where they are coming from and why they feel what they feel. When you can connect with them on this level without them even realizing it, your social skills will then play a role in getting them to open up more and be comfortable around you.

Identifying Your Strengths and Weaknesses

People are quick to talk about strengths, but not everyone likes to admit they have weaknesses. However, the only way you're going to begin developing a great understanding of yourself is by recognizing *both* your strengths and weaknesses together. It isn't going to work if you just acknowledge one, but not the other. Understandably, it's never enjoyable to admit that you have weaknesses. It makes you feel inadequate, and for some people, it feeds into their deep-rooted fear about not being good enough. Others may have a lot of pride, and they simply do not like to admit they have weaknesses because they don't want others to think any less of them.

When you embrace both your strengths and your weaknesses, you begin opening yourself to even greater potential for personal growth. Weaknesses are nothing to be ashamed of. It just means that there are areas for you to work on and you're getting there eventually. This is why self-awareness is so critical.

It puts the power of change in your hands, and you are in control. You are the one who gets to decide if these traits continue to remain weaknesses, or whether you're going to work on them and turn them into strengths.

Everyone should make time to get to know themselves better. The benefits of being more aware of who you are and what makes you tick include:

- **It is the Key to Being Happier.** Chances are if you're not happy, you're mind is going to be too preoccupied to effectively analyze and decipher someone else's body language anyway. The more you understand yourself and your emotions, the happier you will be. It also makes it much easier for you to express your desires.

- **It is the Key to Less Internal Conflict.** Another happiness barrier that many people experience is internal conflict. Understanding yourself allows you to connect to your mind, body, and soul, and when your external actions work in tandem with your internal emotions, the internal struggle that you face becomes significantly less.

- **It is the Key to Tolerance and Understanding.** Analyzing what other people feel is a lot better when you've got tolerance and patience on your side. Your awareness about the emotions and challenges that you face will make you more perceptive towards the plight of others, that they may be going through the same thing you are.

- **It is the Key to More Self-Control.** Knowing yourself also means your values are grounded and you know what your preferences are. It affords you better decision-making abilities because you know what you're willing to put up with, what's acceptable, and what isn't.

- **It is the Key to Succeeding at Work.** Excelling at your job goes beyond just being good at what you do. It involves the way you communicate, the way you relate to others, how well you present yourself and of course, the secret messages that you're revealing through your body language. An employee, for example, may say that they love their job, but their body language could be conveying something completely different. If they aren't self-aware, they won't even realize this is happening. But you know who will notice? The bosses (and your other colleagues who are paying attention).

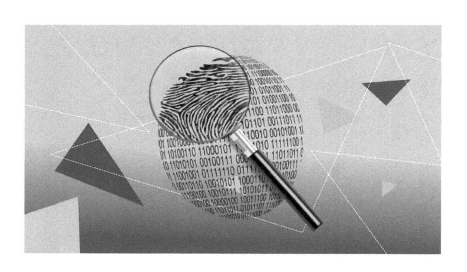

Effective Tools and Strategies to Help You Analyze Yourself

Most people spend far too much time trying to think about what someone else's body language might be saying and not enough time on what their own body language is saying. Becoming too preoccupied with trying to say all the right words makes it easy to forget that your body could be saying something entirely different. If the person you're in a conversation with is perceptive enough, they'll quickly pick up that your body language and your words are not a match.

Consider this scenario, for example. You've just had a long, hard day at work. You're exhausted, drained, and just looking forward to changing into your pajamas and spending some quiet time alone. Then, the phone rings and your best friend wants to talk to you and she sounds upset over the phone. Because you care deeply about your friend, you meet up with them like they requested and agree to talk it out. However, throughout the conversation, you're constantly stifling your yawns, sitting back with your arms crossed over your chest, and constantly checking your watch every couple of minutes while thinking you're being subtle about it. Your friend picks up on these signals and comes to the conclusion that you're either bored or disinterested and they might become even more upset because of that. They leave, visibly upset while you're wondering if you've said the wrong thing. Obviously, you didn't say the wrong words. In fact, you said everything that your friend wanted to hear. Your body was just telling a much louder different story without you even realizing it.

Analyzing yourself is an exercise which is easier than you might think. Start applying these strategies below to help you master your self-reflection process:

- **Taking Note of Your Feelings Daily:** How often do you find yourself noticing your thoughts? Probably not very often up to this point. That is about to change though because your thoughts are a very important part of who you are. These thoughts drive you more than you realize. It shapes your perceptions, your attitudes, and your responses to the people, situation, and circumstances you find yourself embroiled in. Start spending several minutes a day just pausing to notice and monitor what's on your mind. Are the things that you're thinking positive? Negative? Are you empowering yourself and feeling happy? Or stressed, worried, and imagining a lot of worst case scenarios?

- **Writing It Down:** A thought journal can be your greatest asset in your self-awareness reflective exercise. During these moments when you're stopping to monitor your thought process, think about writing them down. Like a daily log journal of your thought process. Write about everything that you're feeling and don't hold back. Your happiness, sadness, frustration, anger, how you reacted today, and what you thought about doing. Anything and everything goes. Each time you've got a thought, put it down.

- **Evaluating Your Thought Patterns:** Another reason why a thought journal comes in handy is that it gives you a chance to look back and evaluate your thought patterns. At the end of the week when you look back on everything you wrote down, what's a common pattern that occurs? What's a train of thought which tends to repeat itself? We've got so many thoughts running through our minds daily that by the end of the day or week, we've forgotten most of the thoughts we had. With a journal, however, you can go back anytime and evaluate everything that went on, anytime. Even something that happened a few months ago.

- **Noting Your Perceptions:** Did you know that the way you perceive people and situations could sometimes lead you to misread things? Or draw on conclusions and assumptions which may not be entirely accurate. For example, if you were having lunch with a friend and you noticed that their body language or facial expression was signaling that they were in a bad mood. Or perhaps feeling irritated and angry. The way you perceive situations could lead you to believe that perhaps she is angry with you or you did something wrong, even though that may not necessarily be the case. When faced with these types of situations, this is where self-reflection once again proves its importance. By analyzing your beliefs, taking note of what you heard, what you saw and what you felt that led you to perceive a situation in a certain way, you will come to realize that situations are often affected a lot by factors which we may not necessarily be aware of.

- **Knowing Your Values:** Your values provide a crucial insight into who you are as a person at the very core. A lot of your current values are based on the experiences that you've been through. Values change as your life experiences change, and rarely do they stay stagnant throughout a person's life. When you can pinpoint and identify each of your values, it brings you one step closer to connecting with yourself. To deepen your understanding and acceptance that this is who you are as a person, and this is what you value in your life. When you know what you want, achieving your goals becomes much easier.

- **Reflect On Your Past Experiences:** Does the way you behave and react to certain situations now a result of your past experiences? A lot of the signals and subconscious messages that we give off is a reflection of our beliefs, values, and attitudes. Even though we don't realize we're doing it. Which is why, it is important to conduct this self-analysis to get to know yourself on a deeper level.

- **Reflecting On Your Self-Esteem:** This is another challenging aspect for many to confront, especially when they suffer from a lack of confidence. What is the status of your health esteem right now? Do you believe you are confident? Worthy? Worthwhile? Or do you struggle with a crippling belief that people are constantly judging you? That you're never good enough? The levels of your self-esteem will affect your body language and the way that you are perceived by others. If you notice when someone is feeling shy or awkward because they're hunched, nervous-looking, and exhibit nervous mannerisms, you can be sure someone else will notice the same thing about you. No matter how well you believe you may be concealing your true feelings.

- **Be Honest with Yourself:** Be completely honest with yourself, even if you may not like what's reflected back at you. You're not going to be doing yourself any favors if you aren't. It's okay, this is an opportunity for you to work on improvements, and there is nothing to be ashamed of if you realize that you have some less than desirable areas that need to be worked on. Even if you try to pretend those shortcomings don't exist, remember that your body isn't capable of telling a complete lie all the time. Someone, somewhere out there is going to be able to analyze your hidden messages. Learning to understand yourself is how you learn to spot the same signals in someone else when you analyze them.

Other Ways of Getting to Know Yourself

Personality tests can be great because they ask questions that you ordinarily would not consider. There are several types of personality tests available, a lot of which can be found online. Some workplaces even provide personality tests for their staff as part of their training programmes. This can be an interesting way of digging even deeper to find out what you're made of.

While initially, these personality tests could just seem like an interesting way to pass the time, or even a fun activity to do during work training, but they have more merits than they're given credit for. A lot of employers these days have come to realize the importance of these tests, and some even now incorporate personality test type questions as part of their hiring process. Understanding personalities are how employers find the best fit for their company.

Keen to find out your personality type? Here are some worthwhile tests to consider investing in:

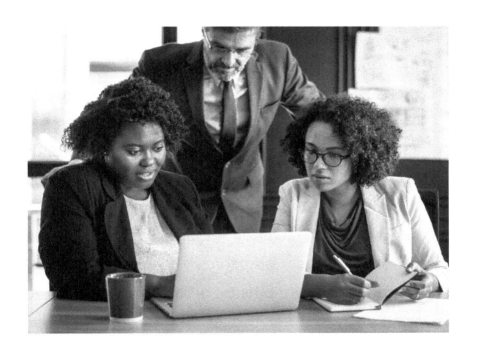

- **Myer-Briggs Type Indicator (MBTI).** Still considered one of the most popular personality tests to this day, the MBTI was created by Isabel Myers and Katherine Briggs based on the ideas of Carl Jung, a psychoanalyst.

- **The Winslow Personality Test.** A test which helps to evaluate 24 personality traits to help you find your strengths. This test is best suited for measuring happiness and success in your career.

- **The DISC Personality Test.** DISC here stands for Dominance, Inducement, Submission, and Compliance. This test was developed based on psychologists Walter Clarke and William Marston's ideas. Companies often rely on this test to gauge the suitability of an employee for a position.

- **The HEXACO Personality Model.** Created in 2000, this personality model measures an individual based on honesty-humility, agreeability, emotionality, conscientiousness, extraversion, and how to open a person is to new experiences.

- **The Revised NEO Personality Inventory Test.** This test was initially developed in the 1970s by McCrae and Costa, and in 2005, it was finalized. Dubbed the NEO-PI-R for short, this test aims to measure what is known as the Big-5 personality qualities. The qualities are, in fact, a little similar to HEXACO's personality model where it namely focuses on neuroticism, agreeability, conscientiousness, extraversion, and how to open a person is to new experiences. Each of these five qualities is accompanied by its own subcategory.

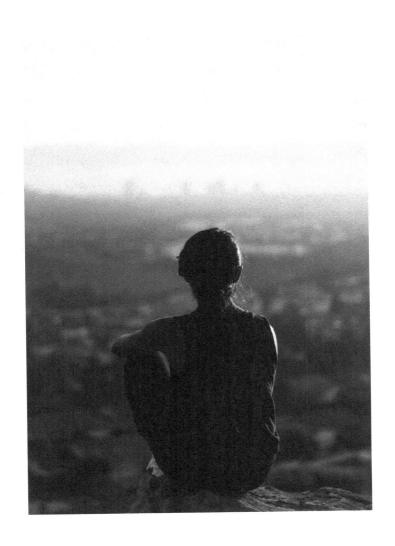

Chapter 2: Body Language and Interpretation

There was once a time when films were silent. If you grew up watching those old, black and white Charlie Chaplin movies, you'll notice how actors like him were the pioneers when it came to sending powerful messages via their body language. After all, it was a *silent* movie, how else were they supposed to let the audience know what was going on? But it's through films like that where we realize just how powerful - and important - body language can be. That our bodies can tell a story so powerful we *still* know what's going on despite the absence of words.

When movies started incorporating sound into them, body language emphasis becomes less and less. Eventually, we came to rely on what we hear and notice less of what someone's body is saying when we watch movies. Silent film actors became obscure, along with essential body language reading skills.

Body language was also studied academically by influential individuals like Charles Darwin, who's published 1872 work on *The Expression of Emotions in Man and Animals* made headway for modern studies on people's facial expressions and body language signals. Since then, there have been many of Darwin's ideas which have been validated by others who have conducted similar research. Albert Mehrabian is another researcher who pioneered the study of body language back in the 1950s. What Mehrabian discovered was that the words we use verbally only had a total impact of 7% on messages; while our vocals had a 38% impact. The vocals here include the inflection of our voices, the tone, and other sounds which may come into play. The biggest message impact, however, came from our nonverbal communication, which was a staggering 55%.

Why It Is Important to Know How to Analyze Others

Actions speak louder than words is not just a saying. Humans didn't always have the ability of speech. Back when the early humans still dwelt in caves, they used body language (and grunting) to communicate what they needed. Their bodies and facial expressions were their primary use of communication. They expressed anger, hunger, fear, love, surprise, and more, all without saying a word. All things considered, speech is still relatively a new way in which we relay our messages, compared to body language which has been present for significantly longer. Because it has been around for as long as it has, our bodies say more about us than our words ever will.

The Benefits of Being Able to Read People

The Significance of Body Language in Deciphering Someone's Emotions

Within the first 30-seconds of meeting someone is when you pretty much start to form your first impressions about them. Even if they don't say a word. How? *Body language.* By observing their mannerisms, facial expressions, the way that they carry themselves, these aspects provide little clues into how they behaved and form your perceptions. Whether they realize it or not, the people around you are constantly transmitting messages with their body, and when you know how to analyze them, what to look for, these messages will become more apparent to you than ever. Even complete strangers around you are conveying secret messages with their body. Are they slouching? Are they standing up tall? Are they fidgeting? Are they frowning? Are they smiling? There are a lot of little clues to look out for.

Body language clues are extremely crucial when trying to decipher someone's innermost thoughts and personality. In many ways, it teaches you to become a human lie detector. Lying with your words is easy enough. We can trick our mind to believe or say anything that we want. Lying with our bodies, on the other hand, is something else entirely. No matter how much you try, you can never get your body to execute a lie perfectly enough. There is something that is always going to give away your true intentions.

Being able to analyze someone's body language is a tremendously powerful skill to possess. It puts you in a position of power because you know something that the other person does not. Body language analysis can also prove to be useful in several job aspects, especially when you're trying to resolve a conflict or a crime. Even when conducting job interviews.

Common Types of Body Language Cues

Body language is the most honest language that we have. Research which has been conducted by those studying this area has discovered that the things that we feel tend to show up in the body first, and only seconds later in the conscious mind. Which means by the time these thoughts have reached your mind, it is often too late because your body may have already given you away.

Leaning to analyze and read someone's body language is about trying to understand and learn what a person's true intentions are. Over the years, we may have become good at masking the way that we feel through our words, but not so much throughout the rest of our body. Did you know that the human brain is hardwired to want to try and read someone else's intention? Or even emotions? That's how the mirroring technique works because we're attempting to mirror the way the person is feeling. To empathize and to share in what we think they may be going through. This is part of our evolution, where we have developed this need out of necessity as part of our survival. When we see someone displaying the fear emotion, we instinctively and immediately know how to react to take the action that is needed.

Assessing body language falls into several categories:

- **Dominant Body Language** is when a person wants to be in charge, in control, or in command of either people or the situation. Individuals who have this desire will usually stand tall with their chest puffed out as a way to express dominance.

- **Aggressive Body Language** is apparent when the person demonstrates body language cues which are perceived as threatening.

- **Emotional Body Language** is displayed when an individual is being heavily influenced by their emotions at the moment.

- **Attentive Body Language** is evident when the person is engaged or interested in their surroundings or people.

- **Boredom** is represented in body language which lacks eye contact. Sometimes, this can be followed by repetitive yawning.

- **Defensive Body Language** is demonstrated by those with a desire to protect themselves or withhold information.

- **Closed-Off Body Language** is evident when the person shuts you out through their body language, such as by taking a step or two back away from you or having their arms crossed in front of their chest.

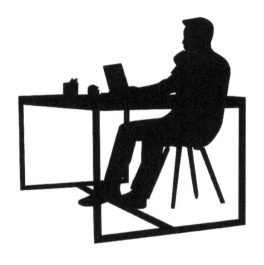

Parts of Your Body That Give Off Signals

Deciphering body language can be complicated. The biggest misconception that we have about body language is that we assume certain gestures have very specific meanings attached to them. When we see a certain gesture, like a person waving their hands, for example, it means that they're definitely saying hello. The truth is body language is ambiguous. Depending on the context, it could have several meanings attached to it. Crossing your arms in front of your chest, for instance, does not necessarily have to mean that you're defensive. It could represent that you're feeling cold, tired, or it could simply mean that you find this position to be the most comfortable for you and that's why you're subconsciously doing it without even giving it a second thought. But to someone who believes that gestures and body language movements mean very specific things, they could misread the situation completely.

The face is a good place to begin if you're attempting to analyze someone via their body language. People like to *think* that they are good at masking and concealing their true feelings, but they're not good enough. Our bodies tend to give us away no matter how hard we try. Our face is where we tend to give off our strongest feelings, even when we try to conceal them. These show up as micro-expressions, which is the sudden "leak" of true emotions which escape the mask we've put on to show the world. Micro-expressions are usually very brief and fleeting, sometimes, lasting for only a split second. But for those who are focused on analyzing body language, a split second is all they need.

Microexpressions are easy to spot when you know what to look for. Let's start with a person's smile, for example. In general, there are five common types of smiles that you could look out for when attempting to analyze someone's body language:

- **A Smile that is Tight-Lipped.** Your first assumption when you see this smile would be that the person is trying to hide their annoyance perhaps. That might be a good guess. But it could hold other meanings to the smile, too. This type of smile - where the lips are stretched tightly across a person's face to the point where it becomes a straight line while still keeping the teeth concealed - could be a signal that the person is attempting to withhold something. Withholding a secret or fighting the urge to speak their mind perhaps because they know it may not be appropriate. This smile can also frequently be spotted on women who are too polite to let someone know they may not be interested. You may also spot this smile among successful, powerful women who may not want to reveal all the secrets to their success. Compare that smile to someone like Richard Branson, for example, who is always spotted with a wide, teeth-baring green and is perfectly happy to divulge helpful information.

—

- **The Twisted Smile.** It's incredible that we are capable of showing two different emotions on either side of our face. But that is exactly what the twisted smile represents. An example of this smile would be where the side of your brain is responsible for raising your left brows, your left cheek, and the left zygomatic muscles. Now, while the right brain is doing this, the left brain is working to do the opposite. The left side of your brain does all the same things the right side does but pulls it in a downward position instead. These are the movements that result in what is known as "the twisted smile". This smile type often makes an appearance when an individual is being sarcastic during an argument or debate. This smile can often be perceived as obnoxious. While a lot of body language signals can represent several possibilities, depending on the context, this smile most often represents sarcasm. That is because this smile is done more deliberately, and it is a reaction that occurs naturally.

- **The Sideways Smile (Looking Up).** You might recognize this smile as a favorite of the late Princess Diana, who was often photographed with the sideways smile while looking up. The person would have their head turned down and facing away while they simultaneously look up at the same time with a smile that is tight-lipped. It is a signal that the person could be secretive, coy, or playful. Men are taken when women perform this smile because it evokes within them feelings of wanting to protect and care for the women. When Princess Diana did it, women liked her and men wanted to protect her. This smile often makes an appearance during the courtship stage of a relationship, too. Prince William now uses this smile often to win the hearts and minds of the people.

- **The Drop Jaw (Smile).** This is another smile which, like the twisted smile, is something that is practiced and done consciously. This smile often reflects that the person is being playful or coy. In this instance, a person simply lowers their jaw (like the name implies) to give off the playful impression.

- **The George Bush Grin.** There's a reason while this type of smile was dubbed the George Bush grin, after the former president. That's because he seemed to have a smirk on his face that was almost permanent. The late American anthropologist, Ray Birdwhistell, discovered that smiling amongst the middle-class was found occurring more frequently amongst residents of Nashville, Atlantan, Louisville, and Memphis. But most of all in Texas, where Texans notably smiled more than other American. Texans were so accustomed to smiling that if someone wasn't smiling, someone might assume or wonder if they were angry or upset about something. Contrast this with New Yorkers, for example, who are accustomed to *not* smiling as often that when you spot a smiling person, you might be inclined to ask if something is funny.

Another area you want to pay close attention to is a person's eyes. If someone is avoiding eye contact, there's a strong possibility their uncomfortable, disinterested, nervous, or bored. If their pupils are dilated, it's safe to say that they are comfortable, perhaps, even like you. If they're blinking far too much (in an unnatural way), there's a strong possibility they may not be entirely honest with you. If they look to the left, they could be recalling a genuine memory, and if they look to the right, it could be a sign that they're trying to make something up.

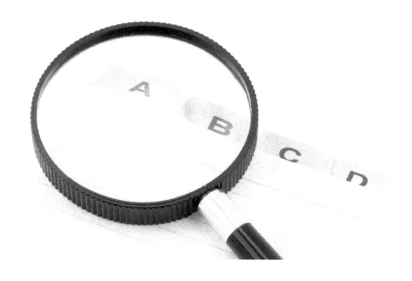

The jaw area is also another good indicator of how a person feels. The next time you're talking to someone, take a quick look at their jaw. Is it clenched? Or relaxed? If you notice their neck muscles may be a little tense, they're giving off signs that they are experiencing a considerable amount of discomfort. They could subconsciously be signaling that they don't want to be a part of this conversation. Or that they may be feeling tense and stressed about something on their minds. Even if what they are telling you with their words may not be conveying that.

Bodily gestures can also be interpreted differently. Here are some of the common body language gestures that you might notice when you start to analyze someone:

- **Having One or Both Arms across Your Body.**
  This is among the most common, universally used body language gestures. As we've already established, having the arms folded across the chest could mean several different things. This gesture is learned by us, even as young children. If you observed children, they tend to hide behind objects when they perceive someone - or something - as a "threat". As adults, of course, it

is deemed unacceptable to run and hide behind an object the way that children do, and therefore, we've turned to fold our arms across our chest. The arms act as a "protective barrier". It is our minds and our bodies unconsciously protecting ourselves from what we believed to be undesirable situations. However, we already know by now that the arms folded gesture could mean several things. It could be a signal that someone is feeling nervous, anxious, defensive, angry, impatient, or perhaps none of the above and they could simply find this position natural and comfortable.

- **Having Both Arms Folded Across Your Chest.** The position of having both arms folded directly across your chest could also hold several meanings. Some people do it because they feel comfortable, while others do it because, on the inside, they feel negatively towards the person or situation. Both arms directly folded across the chest is often perceived to be less than welcoming, and it could put others off because they assume that you're either angry or closed-off to them or your situation. This body language gesture is off-putting to many because it sends the signal that you either do not want to be involved or do not want to participate. It makes those who adopt this stance seem unapproachable. It appears almost as if you were trying to set up a barrier between yourself and the other person.

The way that a person gestures with their hands is another intriguing way of analyzing what emotions or thoughts they may be experiencing. Here are some commonly used hand gestures that depict the following general meanings:

- **Running fingers through the hair -** Uncertain, unsure, or trying to think.

- **Rubbing the brow -** Worried or doubtful.

- **Rubbing the eyes -** Fatigued.

- **Rubbing the ears -** Rubbing behind the ears is an indication the person fears being misunderstood or that they don't understand.

- **Touching the earlobe -** Seeking comfort.

- **Scratching the head -** Deep in thought or confusion (depending on the context).

- **Covering the mouth -** An indication of dishonesty, or that the person does not entirely believe what they are being told. Sometimes, it indicates the person could be thinking about something (depending on the context).

- **Placing index finger on the temple -** Thinking.

- **Touching the Nose -** Associated with lying or feeling pressured.

- **Holding the lips -** An indication of greed.

- **Chin stroking -** Thinking.

- **Outstretched arms -** If this is done with the palms open, it is an indication of the person's openness.

- **Palms facing down -** Confidence, rigidness, or a sense of authority.

How Much Can You Fake It?

Now, humans are capable of choosing the gestures and mannerisms which we want to emit during a speech, for example, or when you're commandeering a meeting. You get to choose the way you project yourself, the hand gestures you want to make, and the stance you want to take while you're speaking. While you're doing all this though, your body is - at the same time - giving out signals which you're not even conscious about. These unconscious emotions are a projection of what you're feeling on the inside.

These gestures may be small and fleeting, but make no mistake that they are still as powerful. The Facial Action Coding System - known as FACS - was developed in 1970 by W.V. Friesen and Paul Ekman. FACS is used to conduct several functions, which include describing, measuring, and interpreting an individual's facial mannerisms and behaviors. FACS was designed to pick up on even the slightest, tiniest facial muscle contractions and movements. It then takes the data and determines which category the facial action that it detected best fits into. What makes FACS so powerful is that it is able to pick up and detect movements and expressions which we may miss with the naked eye. It is a useful device which is often used by those who research human behavior, those working in law enforcement, and even film animators.

There may be times when you may want to conceal how you genuinely feel or even what you may be thinking about. We don't want everyone else to know what's happening on the inside. In that sense, yes, we are able to fake it to a certain extent. But our bodies have a mind of their own. No matter how hard we may try to conceal or consciously control it, your body will still give away tiny little signs and signals that the message you're conveying may not be entirely accurate. To the untrained eye, you may be able to pass off that everything is okay. To those who know what to look out for, they are able to spot signals that everything may not be as it seems.

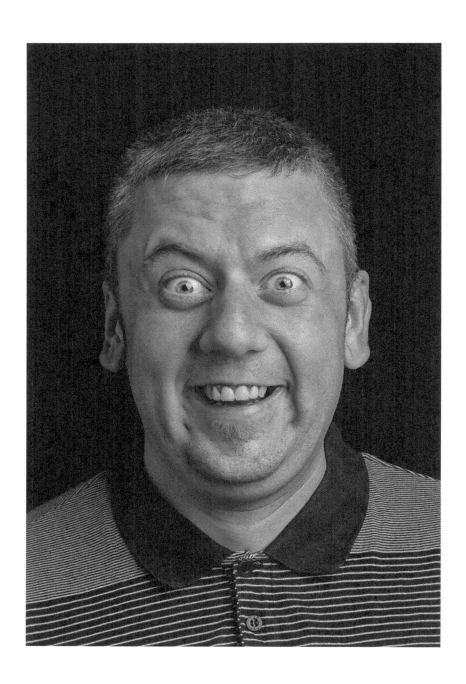

Chapter 3: Non-verbal Communication

Communication seems like it should be a fairly straightforward process. However, nothing could be further from the truth. It's not just about interpreting and understanding what someone is trying to tell you with their words. It is also about all the other dynamics that are going on, what else the person is saying with their body, whether their verbal message is something that should be taken at face value, or if there is something more which needs to be taken into account. That's the whole point of learning how to analyze people because you're now trying to decipher the hidden meaning. Trying to discover what it is that they are not necessarily telling you right now.

Verbal vs. Non-Verbal

When a person uses language and sound to convey their messages and intentions that is a form of *verbal* communication. Verbal communication is defined as a channel by which people use to express their ideas, concepts, and desires. This form of communication is extremely crucial in several settings including work, home, and everyday life. It is how we teach and how we learn, and we use this form of communication more than any other in our daily survival.

The written word is also associated with the act of verbal communication. When we read the words in front of us, we are mentally repeating them to ourselves in our minds. Sometimes, we may even say it out loud. Verbal communication, therefore, involves *both* sound and the written word. Words are the form of communication by which humans have used to exchange their thoughts and messages, especially when they are not in a face-to-face setting.

One example of verbal communication involves public speaking. This is where communication is conducted and carried out verbally to groups of audiences. Another is interpersonal communication, and this involves a group of people who may be simultaneously listening and talking. Other examples of verbal communication include your everyday conversations with your friends, family members, co-workers, clients, and even random strangers you happen to meet as you go about your day.

Verbal communication matters because it is our primary way of conveying our messages. We rely on this method of communication to:

- Inform, inquire, discuss, argue, and spread information and ideas.
- Teach others and learn from them
- Bond and build relationships
- Achieve our desired outcomes
- Work together as a team or group with others towards achieving a common goal

Nonverbal communication, on the other hand, relies on other forms of communication which do not involve the use of words or sounds. This is the category which body language falls into. When we use gestures, body movements, and facial expressions to convey our intent, which is a form of nonverbal communication. Does nonverbal communication matter as much as verbal communication?

Yes, it does. Perhaps even more.

It cannot be stressed enough just how important it is to make a good first impression. One example of where first impressions are absolutely critical is during a job interview. From the minute you walk into the room and even before you have uttered your first word, you are communicating with your employer in a nonverbal manner. Your posture, facial expression, and even the gestures that you make are going to be the clues that your employer is looking for when they assess you. The same thing goes when you're conducting important business or client meetings. The impression that you leave people with can be a big deciding factor in determining the outcome of your success. Saying all the right words, but with the wrong body language, is not going to get you the desired results that you seek.

What You See vs. What You Hear

From the moment you first meet someone, they leave an impression on you. What kind of impression depends on what they convey with their body language. Learning how to analyze someone is about matching what you currently see and hear in the social setting you find yourself in, and then drawing your own probably conclusions. The human brain tends to only see what we want to see, and you now need to learn to push past those boundaries if you want to truly learn the hidden messages which a person gives away with their subtle body signals and movements.

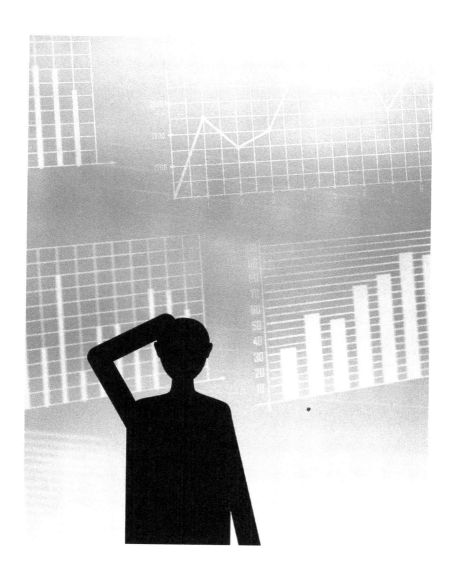

How well do you think you're able to spot contradicting messages right now? Body language is such a fascinating subject area. It is like unraveling a puzzle as you search for hidden clues and meanings to what you see and hear. Politicians are a good place to start practicing your body analysis skills. Politicians are fascinating because there are some who have been guilty of saying that they believe in something which isn't necessarily true. They often pretend to be someone that they are not. As a result, these individuals spend a lot of their time trying to dodge uncomfortable questions, lying, pretending, and presenting a facade to the public to survive. It is their body language which eventually trips them up and reveals telling clues that all may not necessarily be as it seems.

Types of Nonverbal Communication

Communication is the overall concept. To be effective at it, you must be able to communicate clearly with both your words and your body language. In fact, the two should be in sync with one another, because that is when you send some of your most powerful messages across to the recipient – by combining the power of the spoken word with the equally formidable power of body language.

Some examples of the ways in which we communicate nonverbally include:

- **Facial Expressions -** This is responsible for a large part of what we communicate nonverbally. A smile or a frown can be more powerful than several words strung together. Since the face is often the first part of you that people will notice, even before they hear what you have to say, your facial expressions are your strongest nonverbal contact point.

- **Gesture -** The deliberate signals and movements which we use when we're speaking is also a form of nonverbal communication. Waving, pointing, and using our fingers as numeric indicator amounts are all ways in which we communicate with the absence of words. A perfect example of how powerful gestures can be is in a courtroom, where lawyers are well known for relying on several nonverbal communication methods and techniques in an attempt to sway opinions to win their case.

- **Posture -** Body language also involves the posture that you present. Someone who is feeling confident, for example, stands tall, straight, and proud to silently communicate to the rest of the world that they are feeling confident. Someone who is self-conscious, shy, and awkward, on the other hand, communicates this through hunched shoulders and folded arms across the chest.

- **Proximity -** How closely you're standing to someone (and vice versa) is also a form of nonverbal communication. Proximity could differ depending on cultures, and when someone is not comfortable being too close to you, there will be body language cues which you can look out for. This includes averting eye contact, folding of the arms across the chest, tapping their fingers or feet, and visibly taking a step or two back away from you.

- **Paralinguistic Communication** - Now, these include all the other facets of nonverbal communication aside from body movements and facial expressions. Paralinguistic refers to the inflection of the vocals, the tone, pitch, timbre, and rhythm of your voice. These fall under nonverbal communication - even though it relates back to speech - because it involves the underlying aspects of what a person is saying. The tone of voice that they use, for example, could carry a very different meaning from the words that they utter. When a person says *I'm fine* but in a clipped, short tone that carries an edge of anger in it, that's a significant clue that indicates the person is, in fact, not fine at all.

- **Touch** - Among the most widely used forms of nonverbal communication is the element of touch. Touching is a powerful move or gesture which is capable of conveying a wide range of emotional messages a person may want to communicate with you. A warm embrace, for example, indicates that the person is happy to see you or happy to have you around. Or that they care for you and they're pleased to see you after a long period of time. A quick, brief hug, on the other hand, communicates that the person is probably uncomfortable with the gesture, the situation, or that the person is uncomfortable being around you.

- **Locomotion -** The amount of movement that takes place during a communication process is a clear indicator of how engaged that person is. Let's say that the person you were speaking to is constantly moving about, fidgeting, pacing, or simply gesturing far too much, it inhibits the opportunity for effective communication to take place.

Why Nonverbal Communication Matters

Nonverbal communication is a powerful element, and therefore, it does hold several advantages to its name that make it stand out more against verbal communication. When used together with verbal communication, it can result in effective communication and relationship building sessions. On its own, nonverbal communication is still a mighty force to contend with.

The ability to analyze others based on their nonverbal communication, therefore, is an important skill because:

- It helps you uncover the hidden meaning that the speaker is conveying, so you can then tailor your responses appropriately to suit the situation and cultivate your desired outcome.

- Being able to accurately assess and analyze another person's body language enhances your empathy and social skills (which thus improves your emotional intelligence levels). By learning how to identify the telling facial clues and body movements, you will be able to reach levels of communication that others are not, simply because you can see what others cannot.

- It is a clue to providing valuable information about what the speaker is not saying with their words.

- It is used to express emotions and empathy in a powerful manner.

- It increases your understanding of the messages that you receive. When used in tandem with verbal communication, both these elements combined can provide a deeper, more meaningful insight into the speaker's message.

- Being able to interpret these nonverbal cues effectively is how you gain the upper hand over the other person. It is a well-known fact that misinterpretations can often lead to disastrous effects, so why not try accurately analyzing body language instead?

- It helps to strengthen your relationships. People tend to feel a connection to those who they believe can "understand" them in a way that others can't. Being able to analyze body language gives you this ability because you can see the clues about what's really going on, even when the other person thinks they haven't said a word about it.

- The right gestures and expressions can be a strong substitute when you don't know the right words to say. Hugging your friend or family member with a tight, loving embrace can communicate your love and support more powerfully than words ever will.

- It can be used to reinforce messages when used in the right way. When giving someone directions, for example, pointing the right path to take reinforces their understanding about what you're trying to tell them.

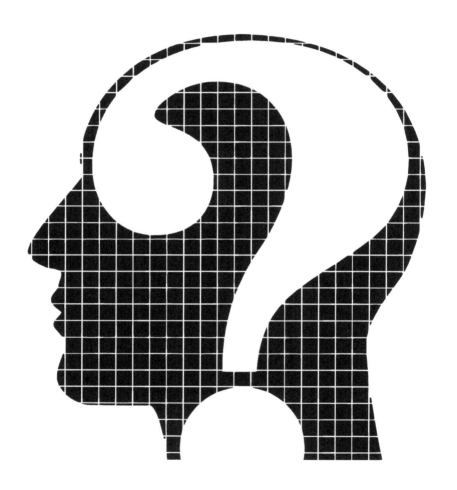

Our non-verbal communication cues are just as important – you might even say of equal importance – to both our verbal and written communication. One cannot exist without the other. To accurately analyze other people, begin by recognizing the importance of *both* these communication forms, not just in others, but in yourself, too. What messages are you transmitting with your body language?

Nonverbal Cues That Convey Confidence at Work

You've got a pretty good idea by now about the nonverbal cues that you need to look for that reveal hidden clues about a person's true desire and intent. But what about the kind of messages *you are communicating with your body language?*

What can you do to give out the right nonverbal signals, especially if you want to achieve success in an environment like your place of work? As important as it is to be able to read and analyze others, we need to make sure that we are also giving out the right messages. Just in case someone is analyzing *you* (and you can be sure that there will be at least one or two people who are reading your clues).

Part of what makes successful individuals so, well, *successful* is the fact that they know how to use both verbal and nonverbal communication to their advantage. Specifically nonverbal communication, which they know can send the strongest messages of all. If you notice, successful individuals often stand tall, straight, and with an air of confidence. They smile, they make eye contact, and they move with intent and purpose. They use carefully chosen gestures during speeches, gestures which have been specifically selected to emphasize the impact of their words to project their messages most effectively.

These individuals know how much nonverbal communication matters that they also know how to position themselves in relation to the people around them. They avoid standing too close because they understand that it could be perceived as either threatening or overwhelming. They also avoid standing too far away because they know it might send the wrong message, that they are feeling distant when it may not be the case. They know how to read their surroundings and anticipate what move another person might make. They have made it a point to understand these skills so well that it has enabled them to succeed in their career.

If you want to start excelling in your career, then effective body language is where you start building your foundation. If there was ever a place where nonverbal communication skills matter the most, it is at the workplace. This is where you are observed the most, especially by your managers and superiors. The most successful people who eventually go on to become leaders and managers at the workplace are the ones who are able to make great impressions on everyone they work with because of how well they communicate. You can be the best at your job in every possible way, but if you don't leave the people around you with a positive impression, there's only so far your knowledge and your skills will take you.

Being confident is an important part of becoming an effective communicator overall. As much as you are busy analyzing the body language of the people around you, there is bound to be at least one or two other people who are *analyzing you.* It is not just the body language of others that matter. Your body language matters, too.

When you interact with others around you at the workplace, the moment you show you are confident, you will find it much easier to hold effective conversations with your colleagues and team members that will result in things getting done. Why? Because they are drawn towards your confident approach. Confident people are not thwarted by challenges, they rise to meet them, and this is what people at work want to follow. Somebody who knows what they are doing and is doing it with confidence.

Remember how our nonverbal cues resonate the most powerful messages of all without uttering a word? That's body language for you. Body language is applicable in the workplace, too, perhaps even more so because this is where it really matters. At work, the way you carry yourself and communicate is just as important as how well you get the job done. To convey confidence nonverbally, you need to start by adopting confident body language whenever you step into your workplace. Do not slouch, do not fold or cross your arms, and do not frown or look sullen. Always be positive and project a warm and welcoming manner. Smile and make eye contact with the people you pass by.

Other ways in which you can project confidence with your body include:

- **Power Poses -** Social psychologist, Amy Cuddy, revealed during her TED Talk in 2012 that power poses can be effective when it comes to appearing and feeling more confident. One example of a confident power pose here involves opening your body and positioning it in such a manner that it seems to occupy more "space". Think of the term *larger than life.* Puff your chest out, roll your shoulders back, and avoid hunching like you're trying to hide away from the world.

- **Observing Your Hand Gestures -** All it takes is for the wrong gestures to be used to convey the wrong message entirely. Being observant about your hand gestures is important in order to portray confidence nonverbally at work. You need to be able to achieve this *without* the use of hand gestures which might be misconstrued the wrong way. When explaining an idea, for example, keep your palms open and your fingers together. This is a universal gesture which communicates openness, trust, cooperation, and acceptance.

- **Holding the Eye Contact** – Maintaining eye contact is one of the most basic rules of effective non-verbal communication. When you engage in eye contact with the person you are speaking to, you are, in effect, showing them that you are interested and keen on hearing what they have to say.

- **Being Aware of Your "Space"**– Ideally, you would want to respect an individual's personal space when you're communicating with them. Spacial awareness is as much a part of the nonverbal communication process as your facial expressions and body posture. Pay close attention to the person you are talking to and watch for signs of discomfort, especially if you are in the office. The minute you notice they are not comfortable with your proximity; take a few steps back to create a comfortable enough space between the two of you.

- **Handshakes Can Be More Revealing Than You Think** – You only get one chance to make a powerful first impression, and nothing leaves quite an impact when meeting someone – especially someone new- than the first handshake. Your handshake will be very revealing to the person on the receiving end, and just one limp, a lackluster handshake is all is needed for that person to be turned-off even before the conversation has had a chance to take off. Think of your handshake as your opening line, the introduction that your body is making. Firm, confident handshakes are a must to convey confidence nonverbally.

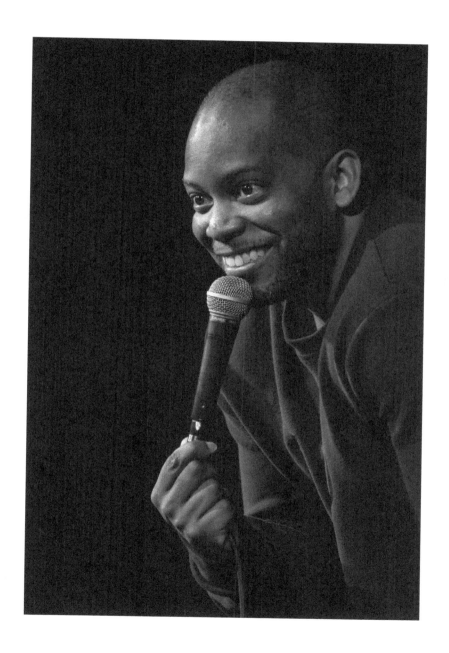

Chapter 4: Asking the Right Questions

Your ability to effectively analyze someone is going to have a big effect on how well you can deal with them. To understand what they feel and to know what they truly mean are important aspects to think about when you're tailoring or adapting your message to communicate in the best possible way. Aside from reading their body language cues and signals, asking the right questions will provide a revealing insight into a person's mind. The right questions can even trigger different body language signals.

The thing about analyzing people is that everybody is different. No two people are ever going to be the same, not even twins. Everyone will come with their own behavior patterns, quirks, and tendencies. Some people look at the floor when they're speaking, some clear their throat, others like to jiggle their legs when they sit cross-legged, and some like to stroke their neck. All these subtle signs are easy to overlook unless you're paying close attention to them and trying to figure out what they mean.

People display different body language cues for a reason. That reason would depend on their true intentions, which only they will know of since reading minds is the one thing that we cannot do. While we may not be able to read minds, we can certainly read bodily signals and that can be used to our advantage, especially when it's paired with the right, subtly probing questions.

What is Effective Questioning?

If you have spent time around children, you will notice that they ask the most intriguing questions. These questions come from sheer curiosity and a genuine desire to find an answer to what they wonder about. They don't even ask complicated or tricky questions. They simply ask questions which are meant to satisfy their curiosity about what's on their mind. They don't guess. They don't assume. *They simply ask.* At some point along the way, we stop asking these questions and this has caused a lot of complications at times in our interaction with others.

Gathering information is something that humans have been doing for as long as we can remember. You might even say that it has become part of the basic activities or tasks that we do as people. Why this need for collecting information? Because humans have been using this technique to help us solve the problems that we encounter, to learn and discover new information, to help out with our decision-making process, and even to understand the people around us better.

When you get better at asking questions, you get better answers. Answers that will help you better analyze the person in front of you. Effective questions are, in a nutshell, purposeful. Questions are effective when they provoke thoughts. They are effective when they are open-ended without being leading. This means that you ask these questions with a very specific intention in mind. You know what you're looking for and what outcome you want to achieve, and you're now using these questions as a technique towards getting what you want. If you wanted to analyze a friend or someone you know, what better way to do it than through a series of questions which are geared towards encouraging them to reveal themselves and their innermost thoughts.

What Makes a Question Powerful?

Meeting new people is one of the most interesting experiences that we go through. Think about it, every partner, husband, wife, best friend, acquaintance, colleague, and significant other once started off as a stranger. It was through effective conversation, asking the right questions, and reading their body language that helped your relationship develop to the stage that it is in right now. You have probably used questioning techniques more often than you realize as you go about your day, it's just that we haven't given much thought to them until now.

When we encounter someone new, we often do not give much thought to the kind of questions that we tend to ask. But, if you were to start consciously *thinking* about your questioning approach and techniques, the outcome of that encounter can be much better than you realize. Questions are powerful methods of getting to know a person because:

- It can be used to discover vital information that could make a tremendous difference in the outcome of a situation.

- It can be used to forge and strengthen new and existing relationships.

- It can be used to seek clarification for deeper understanding, which then helps to minimize the instances of conflicts happening. Assumptions and jumping to conclusions have a higher tendency of occurring when the right questions aren't used appropriately.

- It can help to diffuse conflict and identify the solution that is needed.

- It establishes a baseline for you to begin analyzing someone. This way, your opinions and impressions are formed on more substance rather than just relying on their body language.

- It helps you spot inconsistencies between what the person may be telling you, and what their facial expressions or body language may be revealing. If they're telling you their okay, but you notice a slight frown between their brows or the downward curve of their mouth, asking the right question can help you gently probe what's really going on and help them feel comfortable enough to reveal themselves to you.

- It enables you to direct a person's thoughts in a particular direction.

- It enables you to assess their responses and provide insight into how they may be feeling about a particular subject.

- It provides better clarity about an issue.

- It provides opportunities for open discussion.

Why it is Important to Develop this Skill (Asking the Right Questions)

The heart of effective communication and being able to bond with others lies in the exchange of information. A lack of understanding can act as a significant relationship barrier. Imagine if you were trying to form a bond with someone and they appeared closed-off, distant, or disinterested. Eventually, you would experience frustration because you're not getting through to them, despite your efforts and there is little chance of a relationship blossoming from that encounter.

Which is why asking the right questions is so crucial. The right questions in the right situation can improve your interactions and encounters in monumental ways. You could have the power to control every interaction you encounter if you know how to relate to the person in front of you. You don't have to know them well nor do you have to be their best friend in order to start doing that. By simply asking the right questions, every stranger or acquaintance you come across can be coaxed into revealing what they think and what they feel.

It is impossible to get to know someone in detail by basing it on their answers alone. That's because people lie (and they often do), especially when they want to hide their true intentions which they know others may find less than desirable. Perhaps, they could even tell you what you want to hear to seem more impressive or to avoid conflict. There could be many reasons why a person could resort to hiding their true intentions. Which is why it is important to develop *both* skills of being able to analyze others and ask the right questions which will help to reveal even more hidden clues into their personality.

The human mind is a natural problem solver, and it is through effective questioning that we resolve the challenges that we come up against. Whether those challenges are work-related, or even attempting to learn how to analyze someone, our minds are working even when we don't realize it, to try and make sense of what's in front of us. Body language has become such a fascinating subject of focus in recent years because of it. Once we started to realize that there is more to us than meets the eye (and the words that come out of our mouth), learning how to analyze body language to find the hidden meanings behind words and gestures are more intriguing than ever.

Effective Questioning Techniques

As you are learning how to decipher a person's behavior, there are several important questions which you should bear in mind. These questions are here to help you develop your critical thinking and to enable you to delve deeper into those hidden meanings which lie behind a subtle gesture or facial expression. People are giving off clues and signals every day. All we need to do is watch for it and ask the right questions to encourage them to reveal themselves.

These questions can be utilized as often as you'd like until you have gathered the necessary information required. Enough information at least, which will provide you with enough confidence to say *yes, I know what this person is trying to tell me*. The questions you should be asking yourself when attempting to analyze another person include:

- What body language signals or answers have I observed?
- What do these signals or answers mean?
- What are these signals or answers revealing about them?
- How is this significant to what they are telling me now?

There are two types of questioning techniques which you could turn to. These are known as open-ended and closed-ended questions. When attempting to analyze others, what you're aiming for is *open-ended questions*. That's not to say that closed-ended questions don't have their usefulness (because they do), but open-ended questions will get you further in terms of getting to know someone a lot better. This is because closed-ended questions often only serve to elicit short answers which often put an end to a conversation. When the conversation has ended, how are you going to continue with your analysis of the person?

An open-ended question, on the other hand, is more effective for breaking the ice, especially with strangers or acquaintances. These questions are designed to make a person feel comfortable, and if they are comfortable, they're likely to open up a lot more. This relaxed state is when more body language cues and signals arise because the person is not even thinking about it or consciously trying to control it. Open-ended questions can be an extremely beneficial technique in your quest to analyze others, because:

- It provides the opportunity for developing a conversation.
- It provides the opportunity to find out what the person's opinions or feelings are.
- It provides the opportunity to discover greater details which could influence your responses towards them.
- It provides the opportunity for the person to include more information.
- It provides the opportunity for you to learn something that you did not expect.
- It encourages self-expression in the other person, which then leads to more revealing body language cues and signals.

Contrast that with closed-ended questions, on the other hand, which better serve the following purposes:

- To help you conclude a discussion or conversation.
- To help you make a decision.
- When you want a quick answer.
- When you want to compare answers between several people (such as during a survey)

While these two options may be your primary questioning techniques, there are other methods which can be used if you were looking for more specific answers. Here's a look at some other question techniques which can be employed, depending on whether you need them or not:

- **Funnel Questions:** This is useful if you were looking for answers which were to the point and precise, down to the last detail. You'll see a lot of this questioning method used by detectives when they are attempting to take statements from witnesses to help solve a case. Some examples of funnel questions include *how many people were involved? Who was involved? Can you remember the details of the car? What was the color of the shirt that this person was wearing?* The funnel questioning technique is most effective if you start off with closed-ended questions first, and then slowly lead up to more open-ended questions as the person you're talking to starts to get more comfortable.

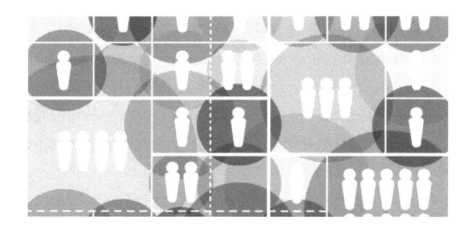

- **Probing Questions:** Another good questioning technique which helps you to clarify answers to ensure that you understand all the facts right. It is an alternative strategy to uncover more detail, too (as most questions are aimed at doing). This is a good method to fall back on when you're trying to gather information out of someone who may be trying their best to avoid revealing something. Probing questions can sometimes be used to help clarify statements by asking such as *when do you need this by? What new information have you received? What exactly do you mean by this?* Using the *who, what, where, when, and why* method is an effective probing question technique to quickly help you uncover the answers that you need.

- **Leading Questions:** This is a good technique when you're trying to direct the person that you're talking to towards your direction of thinking. These types of questions usually fall along the lines of *how late do you think this task will be? How efficient do you think this method is? Do you think we should go with the first option?*

Leading questions should be phrased in such a way that they appear to be personal.

- **Rhetorical Questions:** When you employ this type of questioning technique, you often don't expect them to be accompanied by answers. Rhetorical questions are, in fact, not really questions at all. Instead, they are statements which are phrased in the form of questions. *Didn't John do a marvelous job on the project? Isn't that display absolutely lovely? They have decorated their home wonderfully, haven't they?* These questions are often used to engage the listener and perhaps even draw them towards agreeing with your point of view.

Good Leaders Ask Good Questions

Good leaders know that forging great relationships is one of the cornerstones of success. Without relationships, it would be nearly impossible to succeed because there is only so much you can do on your own. Good leaders know that the path to successful relationships lie in asking the right questions.

The right questions help to build trust, gain understanding, and make the right connections needed to get you one step further. Good leaders are not preoccupied and too focused on having the answers all the time, because *they know* that no one has all the answers all the time. Which is why when they don't know the answer, they turn to *asking the right questions* to get the answers that they see, be it about a situation or a person. Some examples of the right questions to ask include:

- **Easy to Understand Questions -** This one goes without saying. Your questions must be phrased in a manner that is easy for someone else to understand. When preparing your questions, try to put yourself in your receiver's shoes. You may understand what you're trying to accomplish with your questions, but will they? The wrong type of questions, or even questions which are difficult to understand, can quickly shut down a conversation, and that is something that you want to avoid.

- **Specific Questions -** Questions which are too vague or include too much jargon will only make it difficult for others to understand. When they don't understand what you're trying to ask them, they won't be able to provide you with answers which are relevant or accurate. Avoid including too much terminology or unnecessary language in your questions, and instead, focus on keeping them short, succinct, and as precise as possible. Those are the types of questions that good leaders ask.

- **Neutral Questions -** Good leaders steer clear from questions which are either too positive or too negative. Instead, they choose to reframe their questions so that it enables more discussion and exploration. Effective leaders are open-minded and willing to listen to both sides of the argument, and their questions are designed to reflect that neutral stance. This enables them to analyze where all parties involved are coming from, how they feel, and what they think, which then gives these leaders the power to tailor a suitable solution that will keep everyone happy.

- **Questions That Get Right to the Point -** Leaders know how to get right to the point with their questions, and to filter out the information which is unnecessary. Examples of these questions include *why this is happening? How does this affect me or my team? What assumptions are we making in this scenario? What information do we not know yet?*

- **Questions That Inspire Optimism -** Good leaders are advocates for positivity and optimism. They know that negativity can kill dreams and put an end to optimism. What makes them great leaders is that they aspire to inspire optimism and positivity, and one approach to doing this is by asking questions that will inspire imagination, creativity, and rekindle that fire which is capable of driving anyone to success.

- **Questions Which Encourage Teamwork -** Managing a group of people with different personalities and getting them to work together towards a collaborative goal can be a challenge sometimes. Nobody knows this better than leaders do. Which is why, they value the importance of asking the right questions because well-constructed questions can help alleviate the challenges that come with working in a team.

- **Curiosity-Led Questions:** A leader is someone who is always thirsting for knowledge, someone who never stops learning, and someone who is always curious about the world around them. Especially *the people* around them. They let curiosity lead the way when asking questions, and they are not afraid of looking silly or ridiculous. When curiosity is the one leading the charge, it comes from a place of genuine passion to discover answers. This passion, in turn, is what's responsible for asking the right kind of questions that will work to inspire and drive change.

Leadership is about asking questions which can help to do two things - convey who they are as leaders and work to establish credibility. Leaders are not afraid of questions, and they place emphasis on framing their questions well in order to enhance their understanding of what is going on. Oprah Winfrey, Barbara Walters, and Larry King are examples of successful individuals who have mastered the art of asking the right questions which enable them to convey their expertise and what they value.

Good leaders don't just know the right questions to ask, they also know that *listening* is just as important to building relationships and analyzing people. When the person is speaking to you, focus on the word that they are saying instead of concentrating too much on how you're going to respond. If you miss what they're saying, you won't be able to ask the right follow up questions, and this is something that good leaders tend to avoid. Missing out on crucial information leads to misunderstanding, and when you're a leader, you must never be afraid of asking for more clarification if and when it is necessary.

CPSIA information can be obtained
at www.ICGtesting.com
Printed in the USA
BVHW092204080621
609008BV00004B/1106